Table of Contents

Types of dysphagia 2

Causes of dysphagia 5

Symptoms of dysphagia 8

Complications and risk factors of dysphagia 10

How is dysphagia diagnosed? 12

Treatment for dysphagia 15

Dysphagia recipes 21

Types of dysphagia

Swallowing occurs in four phases: oral preparatory, oral, pharyngeal, and esophageal. Swallowing difficulty can be broken down into two categories: oropharyngeal (which includes the first three phases) and esophageal.

Oropharyngeal

Oropharyngeal dysphagia is caused by disorders of the nerves and muscles in the throat. These disorders weaken the muscles, making it difficult for a person to swallow without choking or gagging. The causes of oropharyngeal dysphagia are conditions that primarily affect the nervous system such as:

- multiple sclerosis
- Parkinson's disease
- nerve damage from surgery or radiation therapy
- post-polio syndrome

Oropharyngeal dysphagia can also be caused by esophageal cancer and head or neck cancer. It may be caused by an obstruction in the upper throat, pharynx, or pharyngeal pouches that collect food.

Esophageal

Esophageal dysphagia is the feeling that something is stuck in your throat. This condition is caused by:

- spasms in the lower esophagus, such as diffuse spasms or the inability of the esophageal sphincter to relax

- tightness in the lower esophagus due to an intermittent narrowing of the esophageal ring
- narrowing of the esophagus from growths or scarring
- foreign bodies lodged in the esophagus or throat
- a swelling or narrowing of the esophagus from inflammation or GERD
- scar tissue in the esophagus due to chronic inflammation or post-radiation treatment

Causes of dysphagia

Normally, the muscles in your throat and esophagus squeeze, or contract, to move food and liquids from your mouth to your stomach without problems. Sometimes, though, food and liquids have trouble getting to your stomach. There are two types of problems that can make it hard for food and liquids to travel down your esophagus:

- The muscles and nerves that help move food through the throat and esophagus are not working right. This can happen if you have:
- Had a stroke or a brain or spinal cord injury.
- Certain problems with your nervous system, such as post-polio syndrome,

multiple sclerosis, muscular dystrophy, or Parkinson's disease.
- An immune system problem that causes swelling (or inflammation) and weakness, such as polymyositis or dermatomyositis.
- Esophageal spasm. This means that the muscles of the esophagus suddenly squeeze. Sometimes this can prevent food from reaching the stomach.
- Scleroderma. In this condition, tissues of the esophagus become hard and narrow. Scleroderma can also make the lower esophageal muscle weak, which may cause food and stomach acid to come back up into your throat and mouth.

Something is blocking your throat or esophagus. This may happen if you have:

- Gastroesophageal reflux disease (GERD). When stomach acid backs up regularly into your esophagus, it can cause ulcers in the esophagus, which can then cause scars to form. These scars can make your esophagus narrower.
- Esophagitis. This is inflammation of the esophagus. This can be caused by different problems, such as GERD or having an infection or getting a pill stuck in the esophagus. It can also be caused by an allergic reaction to food or things in the air.
- Diverticula. These are small sacs in the walls of the esophagus or the throat.
- Esophageal tumors. These growths in the esophagus may be cancerous or not cancerous.

- Masses outside the esophagus, such as lymph nodes, tumors, or bone spurs on the vertebrae that press on your esophagus.

A dry mouth can make dysphagia worse. This is because you may not have enough saliva to help move food out of your mouth and through your esophagus. A dry mouth can be caused by medicines or another health problem.

Symptoms of dysphagia

- Some patients have dysphagia and are unaware of it in these cases, it may go undiagnosed and not be treated, raising the risk of aspiration pneumonia (a lung infection that can develop after accidentally inhaling saliva or food particles). ✗

Undiagnosed dysphagia may also lead to dehydration and malnutrition.

Symptoms linked to dysphagia include:

- Choking when eating.
- Coughing or gagging when swallowing.
- Drooling.
- Food or stomach acid backing up into the throat.
- Recurrent heartburn.
- Hoarseness.
- Sensation of food getting stuck in the throat or chest, or behind the breastbone.
- Unexplained weight loss.
- Bringing food back up (regurgitation).
- Difficulty controlling food in the mouth.

- Difficulty starting the swallowing process.
- Recurrent pneumonia.
- Inability to control saliva in the mouth.
- Patients may feel like "the food has got stuck."

Complications and risk factors of dysphagia

Pneumonia and upper respiratory infections specifically aspiration pneumonia, which can occur if something is swallowed down the "wrong way" and enters the lungs.

Malnutrition — this is especially the case with people who are not aware of their dysphagia and are not being treated for it.

They may simply not be getting enough vital nutrients for good health.

Dehydration — if an individual cannot drink properly, their fluid intake may not be sufficient, leading to dehydration (shortage of water in the body).

Risk factors

The following are risk factors for dysphagia:

Aging. Due to natural aging and normal wear and tear on the esophagus and a greater risk of certain conditions, such as stroke or Parkinson's disease, older adults are at higher risk of swallowing difficulties. But, dysphagia isn't considered a normal sign of aging.

Certain health conditions. People with certain neurological or nervous system disorders are more likely to experience difficulty swallowing.

How is dysphagia diagnosed?

If you are having difficulty swallowing, your doctor will ask questions about your symptoms and examine you. He or she will want to know if you have trouble swallowing solids, liquids, or both. He or she will also want to know where you think foods or liquids are getting stuck, whether and for how long you have had heartburn, and how long you have had difficulty swallowing. He or she may also check your reflexes, muscle strength, and speech. Your doctor may then refer you to one of the following specialists:

- An otolaryngologist, who treats ear, nose, and throat problems
- A gastroenterologist, who treats problems of the digestive system
- A neurologist, who treats problems of the brain, spinal cord, and nervous system
- A speech-language pathologist, who evaluates and treats swallowing problems

To help find the cause of your dysphagia, you may need one or more tests, including:

- X-rays. These provide pictures of your neck or chest.
- A barium swallow. This is an X-ray of the throat and esophagus. Before the X-ray, you will drink a chalky liquid called barium. Barium coats the inside

of your esophagus so that it shows up better on an X-ray.
- Fluoroscopy. This test uses a type of barium swallow that allows your swallowing to be videotaped.
- Laryngoscopy. This test looks at the back of your throat, using either a mirror or a fiber-optic scope.
- Esophagoscopy or upper gastrointestinal endoscopy. During these tests, a thin, flexible instrument called a scope is placed in your mouth and down your throat to look at your esophagus and perhaps your stomach and upper intestines. Sometimes a small piece of tissue is removed for a biopsy. A biopsy is a test that checks for inflammation or cancer cells.
- Manometry. During this test, a small tube is placed down your esophagus.

The tube is attached to a computer that measures the pressure in your esophagus as you swallow.
- pH monitoring, which tests how often acid from the stomach gets into the esophagus and how long it stays there.

Treatment for dysphagia

Treatment depends on the type of dysphagia:

Treatment for oropharyngeal dysphagia (high dysphagia)

Because oropharyngeal dysphagia is often a neurological problem, providing effective treatment is challenging. Patients with

Parkinson's disease may respond well to Parkinson's disease medication.

Swallowing therapy — this will be done with a speech and language therapist. The individual will learn new ways of swallowing properly. Exercises will help improve the muscles and how they respond.

Diet — Some foods and liquids, or combinations of them, are easier to swallow. While eating the easiest-to-swallow foods, it is also important that the patient has a well-balanced diet.

Feeding through a tube — if the patient is at risk of pneumonia, malnutrition, or dehydration they may need to be fed through a nasal tube (nasogastric tube) or PEG (percutaneous endoscopic gastrostomy). PEG tubes are surgically implanted directly into the stomach and pass through a small incision in the abdomen.

Treatment for esophageal dysphagia (low dysphagia)

Surgical intervention is usually required for esophageal dysphagia.

Dilation — if the esophagus needs to be widened (due to a stricture, for example), a small balloon may be inserted and then inflated (it is then removed).

Botulinum toxin (Botox) — commonly used if the muscles in the esophagus have become stiff (achalasia). Botulinum toxin is a strong toxin that can paralyze the stiff muscle, reducing constriction. If the dysphagia is caused by cancer, the patient will be referred to an oncologist for treatment and may need surgical removal of the tumor.

How is it treated?

Your treatment will depend on what is causing your dysphagia. Treatment for dysphagia includes:

- Exercises for your swallowing muscles. If you have a problem with your brain, nerves, or muscles, you may need to do exercises to train your muscles to work together to help you swallow. You may also need to learn how to position your body or how to put food in your mouth to be able to swallow better.
- Changing the foods you eat. Your doctor may tell you to eat certain

foods and liquids to make swallowing easier.
- Dilation. In this treatment, a device is placed down your esophagus to carefully expand any narrow areas of your esophagus. You may need to have the treatment more than once.
- Endoscopy. In some cases, a long, thin scope can be used to remove an object that is stuck in your esophagus.
- Surgery. If you have something blocking your esophagus (such as a tumor or diverticula), you may need surgery to remove it. Surgery is also sometimes used in people who have a problem that affects the lower esophageal muscle (achalasia).
- Medicines. If you have dysphagia related to GERD, heartburn, or esophagitis, prescription medicines

may help prevent stomach acid from entering your esophagus. Infections in your esophagus are often treated with antibiotic medicines.

In rare cases, a person who has severe dysphagia may need a feeding tube because he or she is not able to get enough food and liquids.

Dysphagia recipes

Bread Slice

Ingredients

- 5 slices Bread slice (1 oz)
- ¼ cup Milk
- ThickenUp® Clea

Instructions

- Crumble bread into food processor; add milk and puree until smooth.
- Cover and chill quickly (within 4 hours) to 41°F or below before serving.
- Hold for service at internal temperature of 41°F or below.

- Portion one #20 scoop per serving. If desired, use a spatula to shape puree into a square to resemble a bread slice.
- Portions may also be placed between two pieces of plastic wrap, flattened and frozen to set shape. Thaw bread before serving.

Serving Option: For warm bread, cover and heat to 165°F or above before serving.

Nutrition calculations based on using a 1 oz slice of soft, white bread and 2% milk as liquid

Italian Chicken Puree

INGREDIENTS

- l1/4 cup canned chicken
- 1 1/2 tbsp tomato sauce
- 1/8 tsp salt
- 1/8 tsp pepper
- 1 tsp Italian seasoning

INSTRUCTIONS

- Place all ingredients into a small blender or use the back of a fork to blend ingredients until well incorporated and mixture looks soft.
- Move to bowl and microwave 30 seconds.
- Optional variation: add low-fat cottage cheese or ricotta cheese for a lasagna style meal.

Fortified Custard

Ingredients

- Resource 2.0 fibre HN 250ml
- Cream 300ml
- Vanilla essence 1 tsp.
- Egg yolks 5x
- Castor sugar 1/3 cup

Instructions

- Whisk egg yolks, sugar and gradually add heated milk, cream and vanilla essence stirring constantly and return to heat.
- Remove divide into 6 and cool. Or serve warm

Vegetarian Squash Chili

Ingredients

- 1 tablespoon olive oil
- 1 medium red onion
- 1 1/2 cups bell peppers
- 2 celery stalks
- 1 butternut squash
- 4 small garlic cloves
- 1 tablespoon chili powder
- 2 teaspoons ground cumin
- 2 teaspoons unsweetened cocoa powder
- 1-2 tablespoons chopped chipotle in adobo, depending on how spicy you want your dish to be
- 28 ounces can of diced tomatoes
- 5 cups cooked black beans

- 4 cups vegetable broth (for a richer flavor, replace 1 cup of vegetable broth with 1 cup of brewed coffee)
- Salt and black pepper to taste
- Sour cream, minced chives, and lime wedges for serving

Instructions

- Prepare ingredients: Chop the red onion and the bell peppers. Small dice the celery and set aside with the onion and peppers. Peel the butternut squash, remove seeds, and chop into ½-inch cubes. Mince the garlic cloves. Drain and rinse the black beans. Prepare the coffee, if using, and set aside.
- In a 4-6 quart Dutch oven or stockpot, heat olive oil over medium-high until

shimmering. Saute the onion, bell pepper, celery, and butternut squash until the onions begin to soften, about 7-8 minutes. Once the onions become translucent, reduce the heat to medium-low.
- Add garlic, chili powder, cumin, cocoa powder, and chopped chipotle and cook, stirring regularly, until the spices are fragrant and the vegetables are evenly coated, about 30 seconds.
- Add tomatoes, beans, and vegetable broth (and coffee, if using) and stir to incorporate all the ingredients. Bring the mixture to a boil and then reduce the heat to a simmer, cooking for 30 minutes or until the vegetables are very soft and the liquid has reduced and thickened a bit. Before serving,

season with salt and black pepper to taste.
- To serve, divide the chili between bowls and top with a dollop of sour cream and a sprinkle of chives and lime wedges on the side.

Pureed Vegetable Soups

Ingredients

- 2 tablespoons olive oil
- 1 onion, coarsely chopped
- Coarse salt and ground pepper
- Vegetable of choice, such as butternut squash (see below for quantities and other options)
- 1 can (14.5 ounces) reduced-sodium chicken broth

- 1 to 3 teaspoons fresh lemon juice

Instructions

- Step 1 In a large Dutch oven or pot, heat oil over medium. Add onion. Season with salt; cook, stirring occasionally, until softened, 5 to 7 minutes.
- Step 2 Add vegetable, broth, and enough water (4 to 5 cups) to cover. Bring to a boil; reduce heat to medium, and simmer until vegetable is tender, about 20 minutes.
- Step 3 Working in batches, puree brothand vegetables in a blender untilsmooth, transferring to a clean potas you work. To prevent spattering, fill blender only halfway, and allow heat to escape: Remove cap

from hole in lid, and cover lid firmly with a dish towel. Adjust soups consistency with a little water if necessary. Season with salt, pepper, and lemon juice to taste.

PUREED CLASSIC EGG SALAD

Ingredients

- 2 hard-boiled eggs
- 1 tablespoon reduced-fat mayonnaise
- 1 tablespoon plain Greek-style yogurt
- Salt and pepper to taste

Instructions

- Slice 2 hard-boiled eggs
- Place the egg slices into a food processor
- Chop eggs until there are no longer large pieces
- Add mayonnaise, Greek yogurt, and seasonings to chopped eggs
- Blend well until the egg salad is smooth.

Keto Bread

Ingredients

- 270 gr almond flour
- ½ cup + ⅛ cup freshly ground flax seeds (60 gr)

- 2 tablespoons psyllium husks (10 gr)
- ⅔ cup avocado oil or olive oil
- 7 large organic pasture raised eggs
- ¼ cup water
- 1 tablespoon apple cider vinegar
- 4 teaspoons aluminum and gluten free baking powder (at high altitude use half)
- 1 teaspoon Himalayan sea salt
- Toppings:
- Hulled sesame seeds, poppy seeds, flax seeds, hemp seeds, pumpkin seeds (a mixture of any).

Instructions

- Preheat a convection oven to 350 F (170 C). Grease and line a large loaf pan with parchment paper.
- Process all ingredients in Thermomix at speed 3 until integrated, scrape

bowl and pour batter into prepared baking pan and sprinkle flax seeds + hemp seeds over.
- Bake in preheated convection oven preferably about 25 mins or until a toothpick comes out clean (don't over bake!). Remove from oven, let cool for 10 mins on a cooling rack. Unmold, cool completely and cut with a serrated knife. This bread keeps for about 1 month frozen in a Ziplock bag.
- It makes the best French toast, toast, sandwich or anything!

LIGHTENED-UP CHICKEN POT PIE

Ingredients

- 1 tbsp. olive oil

- ½ yellow onion, diced
- 2 cloves garlic, minced
- 2 tbsp. all-purpose flour
- ½ c. low-fat milk
- 1 (14 oz) can low-sodium chicken stock
- 1 head cauliflower, steamed and pureed
- 1 large carrot, diced
- 2 stalks celery, sliced
- 1 c. frozen veggies, thawed (peas, green beans, corn etc)
- 1 lb. grilled chicken breast or rotisserie chicken, cubed
- ¼ tsp. dried thyme
- ¼ tsp. dried sage
- ⅛ tsp. cayenne pepper
- salt and pepper to taste
- *
- For the biscuit topping:

- 1 c. all-purpose flour
- ½ c. regular or white whole wheat flour
- 1 tbsp. sugar
- 1 tbsp. baking powder
- ¼ tsp. dried thyme
- ¼ tsp. salt
- ¾ c. low-fat buttermilk*
- 4 tbsp. unsalted butter, cold and cubed
- 2 oz. reduced fat cream cheese, cold

Instructions

- Preheat the oven to 425 degrees.
- In a Dutch oven or large oven-safe pot over medium heat, add the olive oil. Add onion and garlic and sauté until tender and transparent. Add the carrots and celery. Cook for 3-4

minutes. Sprinkle the flour over top and whisk constantly until the flour turns lightly golden in color. Slowly pour in the chicken stock, cauliflower puree, milk and spices, whisk to combine. Raise the heat to medium-high and simmer for 10 minutes. Add the thawed veggies and chicken, simmer for an additional 10 minutes or until thick.

- Meanwhile, to make the biscuit topping, in a large mixing bowl, combine the flours, sugar, baking powder, thyme and salt. Whisk gently to combine. Add the cold cubed butter and cream cheese. With a pastry blender, work until pea-size clumps form. Pour in the buttermilk and mix until the dough becomes moist and no loose pockets of flour

remain. Arrange the dough over the top of the filling by forming palm size balls and placing them ¼ inch apart. Brush the tops of the biscuits with additional buttermilk (totally optional).
- Place in oven and bake for 20 minutes or until the tops of the biscuits turn golden brown. Remove from oven and let stand for 5-10 minutes before serving.

Chef's Salad With Kefir Ranch Recipe

Ingredients

Dressing

- 1 1/2 cups plain kefir
- 1/2 teaspoon dried chives
- 1/2 teaspoon dried parsley
- 1 teaspoon dried dill
- 1 teaspoon garlic powder
- 1 teaspoon onion powder
- 1/2 teaspoon salt
- 1/4 teaspoon ground black pepper

Salad

- 1 head romaine lettuce, chopped
- 2 tablespoons cheddar cheese, diced
- 2 tablespoons smoked turkey breast, sliced

- 2 tablespoons ham, sliced
- 1 large hard-boiled egg, chopped
- 1 green onion, sliced thinly
- 1/2 cup cherry tomatoes, halved
- 1/4 avocado, peeled and diced
- 1/4 cucumber, chopped

Instructions

- To prepare the dressing, whisk together all the dressing ingredients until smooth.
- Refrigerate for at least an hour to allow the flavors to meld.
- To assemble the salad, place all the salad ingredients in a large bowl and drizzle with the ranch dressing.

SWEET POTATO PUREE

INGREDIENTS

- 2 Medium Sweet Potatoes

INSTRUCTIONS

- Preheat oven to 200C / 400F and line a baking tray with baking paper/foil.
- Wash and dry the potatoes. Using a fork, pierce the potatoes several times, on both sides.
- Place in the oven and roast for around 50 mins (checking after 45 mins), or until the potato is wrinkled and tender.
- Allow the sweet potatoes to cool for around 10 minutes, peel the potato

and place the flesh in a food processor. Blend until smooth.

Chile Orange Roasted Salmon

Ingredients

- 1/4 cup white wine
- 10 ounces salmon fillet
- 1 teaspoon chili powder
- 1 teaspoon dried oregano
- 2 cloves garlic minced
- 1 1/2 tablespoons light brown sugar
- 2 tablespoons orange juice
- salt and pepper to taste

Instructions

- Preheat oven to 450 degrees. Lightly spray baking pan with no-stick cooking oil. Pour wine into pan and place salmon on top. Sprinkle chili powder, oregano, garlic, brown sugar, orange juice, salt and pepper on top of fish.
- Bake until just cooked through, about 10 minutes. Cooking time will depend on thickness of your fish.
- Serve with Peach Kiwi Avocado Pepper Salsa

THAI CURRY BUTTERNUT SQUASH SOUP

INGREDIENTS

- 3 tablespoons coconut oil
- 1 sweet onion, diced
- 4 garlic gloves, minced
- 1 teaspoons freshly grated ginger
- 2 tablespoons red curry paste
- 3 cups low-sodium vegetable stock
- 4 cups uncooked butternut squash, (1-inch) cubes
- 1 (14 ounce) can coconut milk
- 1 lime, juiced
- 1/4 teaspoon salt
- 1/4 teaspoon pepper
- 1/2 cup torn fresh cilantro for serving
- 1/3 cup chopped roasted peanuts for serving

INSTRUCTIONS

- Heat a large pot over medium-low heat and add coconut oil. Once it's melted, add in the onions and the garlic with a pinch of salt and stir. Cook until the onions are soft and translucent, about 5 minutes. Add in the ginger and curry paste and stir until it is incorporated. Cook the curry and onion mixture for 5 minutes, stirring occasionally. Pour in the stock and add the squash cubes. Cover the pot and increase the heat to medium. Cook until the squash is soft, about 20 minutes.
- Once the squash is soft, turn off the heat and very carefully pour the entire mixture into a blender. Blend until the soup is smooth and pureed. Pour it back into the pot and turn the heat on

to medium low. Add in the coconut milk, lime juice, salt and pepper, and stir. Cover and cook the soup for 10 minutes until it's completely warm. Taste and season additionally if desired. Serve the soup with a garnish of torn cilantro and crushed peanuts.

CREAMY POTATO SOUP

INGREDIENTS

- 3 Cups Chicken Broth
- 1 Cup Water
- 2 teaspoons Chicken Soup Base
- 5 Large Potatoes, peeled and diced into small bite sized pcs (should come to 5 cups)
- 1 Cup Onion, diced

- 1 teaspoon Minced Garlic
- 3 Tablespoons Butter
- 2 Tablespoons Flour
- 4 Ounces Cream Cheese
- 1/2 Cup Half and Half
- 1 teaspoon Sea Salt
- 1/2 teaspoon Black Pepper
- 2 teaspoons Chives

Instructions

- In a medium sized pot, add the chicken stock, water, chicken base and bring to a boil. Lower the heat to a simmer and add the potatoes. Cook until the potatoes are tender and can be pierced with a fork (10 min)
- Meanwhile, in another pot, add the butter over low/med heat. Once it has melted, add the onions and cook

until soft and translucent stirring often (approx. 5 min). Season with salt and pepper. Add a teaspoon of oil if the onions get too dry. Add the garlic and cook another minute.
- Sprinkle the flour over the butter and cook for 2 minutes.
- Scoop out 3 cups of chicken stock and add into the butter/flour mixture (in 1 cup increments) whisking until combined. Add 3/4 of the potatoes to the pot.
- Using an immersion blender, blend the soup until smooth. Add the remaining potatoes, half and half and cream cheese, stirring until it has all melted and blended.
- Garnish with chives, shredded cheese, bacon bits if desired.

Carrots, Broccoli & Cheese Puree

Ingredients

- 300g potatoes, peeled & chopped
- 1 medium carrot, peeled & sliced
- 75g broccoli florets
- 4 tbsp of your baby's usual milk
- 15g unsalted butter
- 40g Cheddar cheese, grated

Instructions

- Put the potatoes and carrot into a saucepan, cover with boiling water and cook until tender (about 20 minutes).
- Meanwhile, steam the broccoli for about 7 minutes until tender.

Alternatively add broccoli to the potatoes and carrot after about 12 minutes.
- Drain the potato and carrot and mash together with the broccoli, milk, butter and cheese.

Hot, Buttered Cauliflower Puree

Ingredients

- Two 2-pound heads of cauliflower, cored and separated into 2-inch florets
- 2 cups heavy cream
- 1 1/2 sticks unsalted butter

- Salt
- Cayenne pepper

Instructions

- Step 1 Preheat the oven to 325°. In a large pot of boiling salted water, cook the cauliflower florets until tender, about 7 minutes. Drain well. Spread the cauliflower on a large rimmed baking sheet. Bake for about 5 minutes, to dry it out.
- Step 2 In a small saucepan, combine the heavy cream with the butter and bring to a simmer over moderate heat just until the butter is melted.
- Step 3 Working in batches, puree the cauliflower in a blender with the warm cream mixture; transfer the puree to a medium microwave-safe

bowl. Season with salt and cayenne. Just before serving, reheat the puree in the microwave in 1-minute intervals, stirring occasionally.

Luxurious, Buttery Creamed Spinach Recipe

Ingredients

- 2 lbs baby spinach leaves, washed
- ½ cup heavy cream
- 2 oz butter (½ stick)
- ¼ cup grated Parmesan cheese
- Kosher salt and freshly ground black pepper, to taste

Instructions

- In a large, heavy-bottomed pot (such as an enameled Dutch oven), heat the spinach leaves over medium-high heat. You can add a small amount of water to the pot before adding the spinach, but the leaves will steam in their own liquid as they cook. Stir with a wooden spoon to keep everything moving.
- As you cook it, the spinach will soften and turn a bright green color while reducing in volume quite dramatically. This might take 5 to 6 minutes or a bit longer. Plunge the cooked spinach leaves into a large bowl of ice water. This will stop the spinach from cooking and lock in that bright green color. Drain the ice water and squeeze the excess water from the spinach.

Squeezing by hand, a handful at a time is the best way to do this. You can transfer each squeezed handful directly into the bowl of your food processor since the next step will be puréeing it. Meanwhile, heat the cream over medium heat. Let the cream reduce slightly while you're squeezing the spinach. Purée the spinach in a food processor until it's completely smooth. Return the puréed spinach to the pot and add the butter, cream, and cheese. Cook over medium heat, stirring continuously until it's hot. Season to taste with Kosher salt and a generous amount of freshly ground black pepper. Serve right away.

One Pot Veggie Dal

Ingredients

- 3 Tbsp. olive oil
- 1 yellow onion, diced
- 2 diced jalapeño (optional)
- 2 Tbsp. fresh ginger, minced
- 4 cloves garlic, minced
- 1 Tbsp. curry powder
- 1 can (15 oz.) crushed tomatoes
- 1 red bell pepper, diced
- 3 1/2 cups water
- 1 cup lentils, soaked in water for two hours and drained
- 10 oz. fresh spinach, chopped
- 1 tsp. salt
- cilantro for garnish (optional)

Instructions

- In large pot, heat oil and sauté onion, jalapeño (if using), ginger, garlic and curry powder. Combine well and cook until aromatic.
- Add tomatoes and cook for 10 minutes on medium-high heat.
- Stir in water and drained lentils and bring to boil. Reduce heat to low and cook for approximately 30 minutes or until lentils are soft enough to mash (adding more water if necessary to extend the cooking time).
- Add salt and spinach cook until wilted, 1-2 minutes.
- Serve over warm brown rice and garnish with cilantro, optional.

Beef & Barley Soup

Ingredients

- 1 ½ pounds boneless beef sirloin steak
- 2 (14 ounce) cans reduced-sodium beef broth
- 1 (14.5 ounce) can stewed tomatoes
- 3 medium carrots, cut into 1/2-inch slices
- 2 small onions, cut into wedges
- ½ cup regular barley (not quick-cooking)
- ½ cup water
- 1 bay leaf
- 1 teaspoon dried thyme, crushed
- 2 cloves garlic, minced

Instructions

- Step 1
- Trim fat from meat. Cut the meat into 3/4-inch pieces. In a 3 1/2- or 4-quart slow cooker (see Tip), combine the meat, broth, undrained tomatoes, carrots, onions, barley, the water, bay leaf, thyme, and garlic.
- Step 2
- Cover and cook on Low for 9 to 11 hours or on High for 4 1/2 to 5 1/2 hours. Remove and discard the bay leaf.

Chicken and Cheddar Souffle

Ingredients

- Unsalted butter for greasing the souffle dish, plus 1/2 stick (4 tablespoons), at room temperature
- 1/4 cup all-purpose flour
- 1 1/2 cups whole milk, at room temperature
- 1/2 teaspoon ground nutmeg
- Kosher salt and freshly ground black pepper
- 1 1/2 cups shredded mild Cheddar
- 1/2 cup grated Parmesan
- 2 packed cups baby spinach leaves
- 1 store-bought, rotisserie chicken, breast meat only, skinned and cut into 1/2-inch cubes (about 2 cups)

- 6 egg yolks, at room temperature, lightly beaten
- 2 (1/2-inch thick) slices country-style white bread, crusts removed, cut into 1/2-inch cubes
- 6 egg whites, at room temperature

Instructions

- Special equipment: a 2-quart (8-cups) souffle dish
- Arrange an oven rack in the center of the oven. Preheat the oven to 400 degrees F. Butter the bottom and sides of a 2-quart souffle dish. Set aside.
- In a medium saucepan, heat 1/2 stick of butter over medium-low heat. Add the flour and cook, stirring constantly, for 2 minutes. Slowly whisk in the milk

until the mixture is smooth and creamy. Bring the mixture to a simmer and cook, stirring constantly, until the mixture coats the back of a spoon, about 8 to 10 minutes. Stir in the nutmeg and season with salt and pepper, to taste. Remove the pan from the heat and add the cheeses, the spinach, chicken, egg yolks, and bread cubes. Stir until combined (mixture will be thick).

- In a large bowl, using an electric mixer, beat the egg whites at high speed until they hold stiff peaks, about 2 minutes. Stir 1/4 of the egg whites into the chicken mixture. Using a spatula, fold in the remaining egg whites. Spoon the batter into the prepared dish and bake until the souffle is puffed and the top is firm and golden, about 55 to 60 minutes. Remove from the oven and serve immediately.

VELVETY CARROT SOUP

Ingredients

- 2 tablespoons unsalted butter or olive oil
- 1/2 cup chopped onions
- 6 sprigs thyme leaves, leaves removed and coarsely chopped
- 2 pounds carrots, peeled and roughly chopped
- 1/4 cup slivered blanched almonds
- 6 1/2 cups vegetable stock
- Salt and pepper, to taste

- 1/2 cup heavy cream or coconut cream (optional)
- Amaretti cookies, crumbled (optional)
- Shaved pecorino cheese (optional)
- 1/2 cup slivered blanched almonds, toasted (optional)
- Creme fraiche (optional)

Instructions

- In a large stockpot over medium heat, melt the butter. Add onion and thyme, and cook for 10 minutes, until onion is soft and translucent. Add carrots, almonds, and stock. Bring to a boil. Reduce heat and simmer for 25 to 30 minutes, or until carrots are very soft.
- Transfer mixture to a high-speed blender or food processor. An

immersion blender could also be used. Blend in batches until very smooth.
- Strain the mixture in batches through a fine mesh strainer into a bowl. Discard any leftover clumps.
- Once the soup mixture is smooth, mix in cream until blended. Season with salt and pepper to taste. Divide soup among 4 bowls, and garnish with amaretti crumbles, pecorino cheese, toasted almonds, creme fraiche, and extra thyme leaves. Serve warm.

Cheesy Chicken Broccoli Bake

INGREDIENTS

- 1 tbsp. extra-virgin olive oil
- 1 c. small yellow onion, chopped
- 2 cloves garlic, minced
- 1 lb. boneless, skinless chicken breasts, cut into 1-inch pieces
- Kosher salt
- Freshly ground black pepper
- 1 c. white rice
- 2 1/2 c. low-sodium chicken broth, divided
- 1 c. heavy cream
- 2 c. broccoli florets
- 1 c. shredded cheddar
- 1/4 c. panko bread crumbs

Instructions

- In a large oven-safe skillet over medium-high heat, heat oil. Add onion and cook, stirring, until soft, 5 minutes. Add garlic and cook until fragrant, 1 minute more. Add chicken and season with salt and pepper. Cook, stirring occasionally, until golden, about 6 minutes more.
- Stir in rice, heavy cream, and 1 cup of the broth. Bring to a simmer and cook until rice is tender, about 15 minutes. Add remaining 1 1/2 cups broth, broccoli, and cheddar cheese and cook until broccoli is tender and cheese is melty, about 10 minutes.
- Heat broiler. Sprinkle chicken mixture with bread crumbs and season with salt and pepper. Broil until golden and crispy, about 2 minutes.

Made in the USA
Coppell, TX
25 June 2024